Ivermectin A Cure For Covid 19?

Bethany Roberts

Copyright © 2021 Bethany Roberts
All rights reserved.
ISBN: 978-1-312-08740-8

Disclaimer

We have made every effort to make certain that all information is factually correct, comprehensive, and up-to-date. However, this book should not be used as a substitute for the knowledge and expertise of a licensed healthcare professional. You should always consult your doctor or other healthcare professional before taking any medication. The drug information contained herein is subject to change and is not intended to cover all possible uses, directions, precautions, warnings, drug interactions, allergic reactions, or adverse effects. The absence of warnings or other information for a given drug does not indicate that the drug or drug combination is safe, effective, or appropriate for all patients or all specific uses.

Contents

Introduction 6

Ivermectin and Covid-19: how a cheap antiparasitic became political. 8

Is The Left Wing, Anti Trump Element Of US & Globalized Politics, Playing Games With Millions Of Lives? 11

Why might it be used to treat COVID? 17

Front Line Covid 19 Critical Care Alliance. Prevention and Treatment Protocols for Covid 19. 20

Pre-Clinical Studies of Ivermectin's activity against SARS-CoV-2 24

Pre-Clinical studies of ivermectin's anti-inflammatory properties 28

Exposure prophylaxis studies of ivermectin's ability to prevent transmission of COVID-19 29

Clinical studies on the efficacy of Ivermectin in treating mildly ill outpatients 33

Clinical studies of the efficacy of ivermectin in hospitalized patients 36

Ivermectin in post-COVID-19 syndrome 40

Safety of Ivermectin 41

Introduction

Remember to keep all medicines out of the reach of children, never share your medicines with others, and use Ivermectin only for the indication prescribed. Always consult your healthcare provider to ensure the information displayed in this book is relevant to your personal circumstances.

Ivermectin, sold under the brand name Stromectol among others, is a medication that is used to treat parasite infestations. In humans, this includes head lice, scabies, river blindness, strongyloidiasis, trichuriasis, ascariasis, and lymphatic filariasis.

In 1975, Professor Satoshi Omura at the Kitsato institute in Japan isolated an unusual Streptomyces bacterium from the soil near a golf course along the south east coast of Honshu, Japan.

Omura, along with William Campbell, found that the bacterial culture could cure mice infected with the roundworm Heligmosomoides polygyrus.

Campbell isolated the active compounds from the bacterial culture, naming them "avermectins" and the bacterium Streptomyces avermitilis for the compounds' ability to clear mice of worms (Crump and Omura, 2011).

Despite decades of searching around the world, the Japanese microorganism remains the only source of avermectin ever found. Ivermectin, a derivative of avermectin, then proved revolutionary. Originally introduced as a veterinary drug, it soon after made historic impacts in human health, improving the nutrition, general health and wellbeing of billions of people worldwide ever since it was first used to treat Onchocerciasis (river blindness) in humans in 1988.

It proved ideal in many ways, given that it was highly effective, broad-spectrum, safe, well tolerated and could be easily administered (Crump and Omura, 2011).

Although it was used to treat a variety of internal nematode infections, it was most known as the essential mainstay of two global disease elimination campaigns that has nearly eliminated the world of two of its most disfiguring and devastating diseases.

The unprecedented partnership between Merck & Co. Inc., and the Kitasato Institute combined with the aid of international health care organizations has been recognized by many experts as one of the greatest medical accomplishments of the 20th century.

One example was the decision by Merck & Co to donate ivermectin doses to support the Meztican Donation Program which then provided over 570 million treatments in its first 20 years alone (Tambo et al.). Ivermectins' impacts in controlling Onchocerciasis and Lymphatic filariasis, diseases which blighted the lives of billions of the poor and disadvantaged throughout the tropics, is why its discoverers were awarded the Nobel Prize in Medicine in 2015 and the reason for its inclusion on the WHO's "List of Essential Medicines." Further, it has also been used to successfully overcome several other human diseases and new uses for it are continually being found (Crump and Omura, 2011).

In the intervening years, the effectiveness of ivermectin and its derivatives in treating parasitic worm infections transformed human and veterinary medicine, leading to a Nobel Prize for its discoverers, William C Campbell and Satoshi Ōmura.

Ivermectin and Covid-19: how a cheap antiparasitic became political.

The common antiparasitic ivermectin is being touted as a miracle cure for Covid-19 by doctors and campaigners the world over. Demand for approval of the drug is growing globally – with some countries recommending ivermectin as a treatment for coronavirus patients.

In the year since the Covid-19 pandemic began, various unconventional treatments have been hailed as potential cures for the respiratory virus that has so far claimed over three million lives worldwide.

While the likes of dexamethasone, Gilead's remdesivir and various monoclonal antibody treatments have been granted emergency approval for the treatment of certain hospitalized Covid-19 patients, the availability of these drugs varies wildly around the world, and supplies are particularly scarce in the most resource-limited settings. In these conditions, and with large numbers of new cases still being reported in various countries, the stage is set for some citizens and physicians to improvise with unapproved or off-label remedies.

The drug, which was discovered in 1975 and commercialized in the early 1980s, came into the Covid-19 picture after Australian researchers last year reported it could inhibit in vitro coronavirus replication in large doses.

Commonly used to treat parasites in animals and head lice in humans, the drug has now been permitted as a treatment for Covid-19 patients in several of the worst-hit countries, including Slovakia, the Czech Republic and swathes of Latin America.

The pro-ivermectin campaign has taken a particularly strong hold in South Africa, where coronavirus infection rates are among the worst in the continent and the vaccination programme has yet to cover all of the country's most vulnerable. Some doctors have been prescribing the worm drug to Covid-19 patients, claiming anecdotally that it alleviates virus symptoms.

Ivermectin–Widely Used To Treat Covid-19 Despite Being Unproven Is Being Studied In The U.K. As A Potential Treatment

The University of Oxford announced it is investigating antiparasitic drug ivermectin as a possible treatment for Covid-19, a trial that could finally resolve questions over the controversial medicine which has been widely promoted around the world despite warnings from regulators and a lack of data supporting its use.

Ivermectin will be assessed as part of the U.K. government-backed Principle study, which assesses non-hospital treatments against Covid-19 and is a large-scale randomized control trial widely considered the "gold standard" in evaluating a medicine's effectiveness.

While studies have shown ivermectin to inhibit virus replication in a lab, studies in people have been more limited and have not conclusively demonstrated the drug's effectiveness or safety for the purpose of treating Covid-19.

The medicine has a good safety profile and is used widely around the world to treat parasitic infections like river blindness.

Professor Chris Butler, one of the study's lead investigators, said the group hopes "to generate robust evidence to determine how effective the treatment is against Covid-19, and whether there are benefits or harms associated with its use."

Ivermectin is the seventh treatment to be tested in the Principle trial, two of which—the antibiotics azithromycin and doxycycline—were found to be generally ineffective in January and one—an inhaled steroid, budesonide—was found to be effective at reducing recovery time in April.

Dr. Stephen Griffin, an associate professor at the University of Leeds, said the trial should finally provide an answer to questions over whether ivermectin should be used as a drug targeting Covid-19. "Much like hydroxychloroquine before, there has been a considerable amount of off-label use of this drug," primarily based on studies of the virus in laboratory settings, not people, and using safety data from its widespread use as an antiparasitic, where much lower doses are normally used. Griffin added: "The danger with such off-label use is that… the drug becomes driven by specific interest groups or proponents of non-conventional treatments and becomes politicized." The Principle study should help "resolve ongoing controversy," Griffin said.

But with the ongoing Political weaponization of Covid cures, it may be wise to not hold your breath.

As the search continues for treatments for COVID-19, the results from a number of studies have led to changes in the advice on which drugs to give people who are suffering from the disease.

The European Medicines Agency and the United States National Institutes of Health have recently stated that one previously promising treatment – the antiparasitic drug, ivermectin – is not recommended for use in routine management of COVID-19 patients.

Despite these decisions, support for ivermectin has been circulating on social media and in WhatsApp groups, with rumors abounding that the drug is being blocked on purpose. Some have dubbed it the "new hydroxychloroquine".

Is The Left Wing, Anti Trump Element Of US & Globalized Politics, Playing Games With Millions Of Lives?

In 2020, the President of the United States of America made a claim that Hydroxychloroquine could be used as a treatment for Covid 19.

The FDA authorized the emergency use of hydroxychloroquine in March 2020. A week later Donald Trump endorsed the drug as a potential Covid-19 treatment and the government stockpiled millions of doses. The President only made his statement after being briefed by the FDA that it was indeed a 'game changer'.

The 'Left Wing' element of US politics and news, then quickly jumped on this statement to use this as a weapon against the former President and any simple drug that worked including ivermectin was attacked.

A study was released by infectious-disease researchers in New Jersey. The researchers studied 255 patients at Saint Barnabas Medical Center in Livingston, N.J., during the early months of the pandemic. They conclude that a combination of hydroxychloroquine and azithromycin at certain levels translates to "a survival rate 2.9 times the other patients."

Trump himself recently released a list of things "they are now admitting I was right about" that included, with no qualification, "Hydroxychloroquine works."

Hydroxychloroquine, the malaria drug touted as a "game changer" magical Covid-19 cure by former US President Donald Trump in 2020, has been found effective in a prophylactic study published in the Journal of The Association of Physicians of India.

Hydroxychloroquine may have become politicized in the US but India uses it widely.

"It's the politicization of this medicine by the mainstream media and portions of the medical community that somehow made this a battle between President (Donald) Trump and them, and created this undue fear and hysteria over a drug, a medicine that has been used for over 60 years relatively safely and is regularly prescribed to pregnant women if they are going to a malaria zone," White House Office of Trade and Manufacturing Policy Director Peter Navarro told reporters.

"The idea that this is a dangerous drug is just silly, but if you ask the American people based on the media's coverage of it, that is kind of the state of play right now," he said.

Navarro said four doctors at the Detroit Hospital System filed a request for emergency use authorization for hydroxychloroquine. The request was for three things;

"One, for early treatment use in a hospital setting. Number two, treatment between a doctor and his patient in an outpatient setting. Three, not just as a therapeutic but also as a possible prophylaxis for preventative use," he said.

This request to the FDA comes on the heels of the publication of their study in the Journal of Infectious Diseases last week that showed an astonishing 50 per cent reduction in the mortality rate for patients taking hydroxychloroquine, Navarro said.

"Give hydroxy a chance, and please don't contribute to hydroxy hysteria because if it's prescribed under the supervision of a doctor, the odds that it can harm you are way, way smaller than the odds that it can help you," Navarro said.

"This has become highly politicized, but India uses this widely for prophylaxis. There are a number of studies which point to this actually working," Navarro said.

The official said if he were to show any kind of symptoms, he would first ask his doctor whether hydroxychloroquine is appropriate. "And then I wouldn't hesitate to take it," he said.

He said if one looks at the 14-day arc of the virus from the beginning of symptoms, the first seven days are critical: when a person may have fever, dry cough, possibly a profound sense of fatigue.

"At that point, your lungs are still intact, and the virus is not appreciably spread to the rest of your organs. Hydroxychloroquine, based on the science in articles like the one that originally appeared in 2005 in the Journal of Virology, works in a therapeutic way by raising the alkalinity of your cells which slows the replication of the virus and also can kill the virus," he said.

"It also has an anti-inflammatory effect, which is why it is used for rheumatoid arthritis, and the drug can, therefore, also help manage what is called the cytokine storm", he said

In the competition between East and West over global governance models, it seems Asian countries may be emerging as the winners when it comes to health governance. Asian countries overall have fared better in managing the Covid-19 pandemic, with lower mortality rate which are attributed to Asian culture, climate, demographics, prior experience with SARS and MERS coronaviruses, and use of antimalarial drug hydroxychloroquine. Given the more successful mitigation models compared to their western counterparts, Asian countries appear likely to continue heeding their own judgement and guidelines for pandemic management rather than deferring to Western models.

On the issue of pandemic management, currently East Asian and South Asian countries enjoy comparative lower mortality rate for Covid-19 than western countries.

Taiwan, now touted as the gold standard for pandemic management, has a population of 23.7 million people but only seven deaths.

Vietnam has registered zero deaths with a population of 95.5 million, while South Korea (population: 51 million) has lost 300 and Japan (population: 126 million) has lost 1001.

In contrast, the US (population: 328 million) has lost 154,000 while the UK (population: 66 million) has lost 45,961. Italy (population 60 million) has lost 35,121, Spain (population: 47 million) has lost 28,443 while France (population: 67 million) has lost 30,238 and Germany (population: 83 million) has lost 9,217.

In order to control for population variance across countries, as measured by case-fatality-rate (CFR) per 100,000 people, Asian countries still rank lower in the CFR vis-à-vis Western countries.

According to Johns Hopkins University, European countries have the highest CFR rate in double digits with UK at 15.2% followed by Belgium (14.6%), Italy (14.2%), France (13.7%), Spain (10.1%), and Germany and US at 4.4% and 3.4% respectively.

In Asia, CFR is at single digits with China is at 5.3% followed by Japan (3%), India (2.2%), South Korea (2.1%), Malaysia (1.4%), Taiwan (1.5%) and Singapore (0.1%).

There have been debates over the reason for this discrepancy, ranging from Asian culture of wearing masks, climate contrasts, genetic differences, younger demographic, and previous experience with the SARS coronavirus and MERS coronavirus epidemics that enabled faster responses to the new threat.

Another possible reason is the widespread use of the anti-malarial drug Hydroxychloroquine (HCQ), which has somehow become a political football in the West.

HCQ is an anti-viral drug sold under the brand name Plaquenil as well as a generic medicine. It has been around for 60 years, and is often used to treat malaria, lupus, rheumatoid arthritis, and other autoimmune diseases.

In 2005, US National Institute of Health (NIH) reported in its journal Virology that chloroquine, a more toxic form of hydroxychloroquine, was effective in preventing the spread of Covid-19's predecessor SARS.7

Covid-19 is the novel SARS Coronavirus 2 (SARS-CoV-2), which is genetically closely related to the SARS Coronavirus (SARS-CoV) from 2002.

Authored by Martin J Vincent, Eric Bergeron, Suzanne Benjannet, Bobbie R Erickson, Pierre E Rollin, Thomas G Ksiazek, Nabil G Seidah, and Stuart T Nichol, the study concluded that "Favorable inhibition of virus spread was observed when the cells were either treated with chloroquine prior to or after SARS CoV infection", and this appears to be supported by health experts in Asian countries.

For example, India and Indonesia stand by the antimalarials, with Indian Council for Medical Research (ICMR) arguing they found no evidence the drug caused harm as a prophylaxis and encouraging HCQ as a preventive treatment for its medical workers. Indonesian doctors also use the drug to treat all Covid-19 patients and has ramped up its production, granting licenses to local manufacturers to produce millions of doses.

In South Korea, Korean Centers for Disease Control and Prevention also used HCQ in combination with an anti-HIV drug to effectively treat Covid-19, as well as in Taiwan for treating mild cases. Likewise, Malaysia found the antimalarial effective in treating early stages of Covid-19 infections. Malaysian Health Director-General Dr. Noor Hisham Abdullah said the off-label use of HCQ managed to delay Covid-19 progression that could have led to low fatality rates in the country.

He divides Covid-19 infections into four stages: the first is testing positive without symptoms; the second stage shows mild symptoms; the third is pneumonia but does not need oxygen; the fourth stage is pneumonia needing oxygen; and the fifth stage is needing ventilator support. In Malaysia, 88% of its Covid-19 cases are in the first two early stages, and Dr. Abdullah observed the impact of HCQ is mainly on Categories 1 and 2 which prevented deterioration into Categories 4 and 5.

It is important to point out that HCQ is not a cure, nor is it an effective treatment for severe case of Covid19. Rather, many Asian countries use it to treat early and mild cases of the virus to prevent it from becoming worse, which according to a recent Henry Ford Hospitals group study of 2,500 patients, show promise it could reduce mortality by about half compared to those not given the drug. The Association of American Physicians and Surgeons (AAPS) seems to share views on the drug's benefits as well.

In light of Asian countries' lower mortality rate and comparative success in Covid-19 management, perhaps this time Western countries could take some lessons learned from their model of health governance.

It may also benefit a seemingly politicized WHO to learn from Taiwan which has emerged as a successful model for managing Covid-19, yet continues to be banned from WHO membership. Given this, in conjunction with WHO's at times contradictory guidance on Covid-19, it appears Asian countries will likely continue to exercise their own judgement when it comes to guidelines for mitigating the pandemic.

Why might it be used to treat COVID?

How did a drug mainly used to treat intestinal parasites in cows come to be of interest to doctors treating humans with COVID-19?

In early 2020, a paper was made public (before it was reviewed by other scientists) which showed ivermectin suppresses the replication of the SARS-CoV-2 virus, which causes COVID-19, under laboratory conditions. This was one of many studies over the past 50 years to show that the antiparasitic drug could also have antiviral uses.

There appear to be two key ways in which the drug could prevent coronavirus replication. First, it could prevent the virus from suppressing our cells' natural antiviral responses. Second, it's possible the drug prevents the "spike" protein on the surface of the virus from binding to the receptors that allow it to enter our cells. Along with the anti-inflammatory actions apparent from ivermectin's efficacy in rosacea, these may point towards useful effects in a viral disease that causes significant inflammation.

These initial findings were used as the basis of numerous recommendations for ivermectin's use to treat COVID-19, particularly in Latin America, which were later retracted.

Why is it controversial?

Since then, there have been numerous studies into ivermectin as a potential treatment for COVID-19.

In late 2020, a research group in India was able to summarize the results of four small studies of ivermectin as an add-on treatment in COVID-19 patients. This review showed a statistically significant improvement in survival among patients who received ivermectin in addition to other treatments.

But the authors stated clearly that the quality of the evidence was low and that the findings should be treated with caution. As is frequently the case for reviews of multiple small studies, the paper suggested that further trials were needed to determine whether ivermectin was indeed clinically effective.

A controversy subsequently blew up over an article by the Front Line COVID-19 Critical Care Alliance, a group of doctors and researchers that lobbies for the use of ivermectin.

Critical Care Alliance regard ivermectin as a core medication in the prevention and treatment of COVID-19. For comprehensive information on ivermectin please refer to our Review of the Emerging Evidence Supporting the Use of Ivermectin in the Prophylaxis and Treatment of COVID-19 and the included references.

A more recent paper, Meta-analysis of Randomized Trials of Ivermectin to treat SARS-CoV-2 Infection was accepted for publication July 6, 2021, by Oxford University Press on behalf of the Infectious Diseases Society of America. This study was done by Dr. Andrew Hill and the team that researched ivermectin's efficacy in COVID-19 treatment for the WHO.

The data is overwhelmingly positive and was discussed in detail by Dr. Pierre Kory on the FLCCC's July 7, 2021, Weekly Update. Another recent paper, Ivermectin for Prevention and Treatment of COVID-19 Infection: A Systematic Review, Meta-analysis, and Trial Sequential Analysis to Inform Clinical Guidelines was published online June 17, 2021, by the American Journal of Therapeutics. It concludes, "Moderate-certainty evidence finds that large reductions in COVID-19 deaths are possible using ivermectin. Using ivermectin early in the clinical course may reduce numbers progressing to severe disease. The apparent safety and low cost suggest that ivermectin is likely to have a significant impact on the SARS-CoV-2 pandemic globally."

These following contain the scientific rationale that justifies the use of ivermectin in COVID-19.

Ivermectin is a well-known, FDA-approved anti-parasite drug that has been used successfully for more than four decades to treat onchocerciasis "river blindness" and other parasitic diseases. It is one of the safest drugs known.

It is on the WHO's list of essential medicines, has been given 3.7 billion times around the globe, and has won the Nobel prize for its global and historic impacts in eradicating endemic parasitic infections in many parts of the world. Our medical discovery of a rapidly growing published medical evidence base, demonstrating ivermectin's unique and highly potent ability to inhibit SARS-CoV-2 replication and to suppress inflammation, prompted our team to use ivermectin for prevention and treatment in all stages of COVID-19.

Ivermectin is not yet FDA-approved for the treatment of COVID-19, but on Jan 14, 2021, the NIH changed their recommendation for the use of ivermectin in COVID-19 from "against" to "neutral".

IVERMECTIN FOR COVID-19
60 TRIALS, 574 SCIENTISTS, 21,814 PATIENTS
30 RANDOMIZED CONTROLLED TRIALS

85% IMPROVEMENT IN 13 PROPHYLAXIS TRIALS RR 0.15 [0.08-0.25]
74% IMPROVEMENT IN 26 EARLY TREATMENT TRIALS RR 0.26 [0.16-0.43]
43% IMPROVEMENT IN 21 LATE TREATMENT TRIALS RR 0.57 [0.44-0.74]
67% IMPROVEMENT IN 23 MORTALITY RESULTS RR 0.33 [0.21-0.51]
60% IMPROVEMENT IN 30 RANDOMIZED CONTROLLED TRIALS RR 0.40 [0.28-0.57]
SUMMARY OF RESULTS REPORTED IN IVERMECTIN TRIALS FOR COVID-19. 07/20/21. IVMMETA.COM

Front Line Covid 19 Critical Care Alliance. Prevention and Treatment Protocols for Covid 19.

Summary of the Clinical Trials Evidence for Ivermectin in COVID-19

Ivermectin, an anti-parasitic medicine whose discovery won the Nobel Prize in 2015, has proven, highly potent, anti-viral and anti-inflammatory properties in laboratory studies. In the past 4 months, numerous, controlled clinical trials from multiple centers and countries worldwide are reporting consistent, large improvements in COVID-19 patient outcomes when treated with ivermectin. Our comprehensive scientific review of these referenced trials can be found on the Open Science Foundation pre-print server here: https://osf.io/wx3zn/.

Properties of Ivermectin

1) Ivermectin inhibits the replication of many viruses, including SARS-CoV-2, influenza, and others;
2) Ivermectin has potent anti-inflammatory properties with multiple mechanisms of inhibition;
3) Ivermectin diminishes viral load and protects against organ damage in animal models;
4) Ivermectin prevents transmission of COVID-19 when taken either pre- or post-exposure;
5) Ivermectin hastens recovery and decreases hospitalization and mortality in patients with COVID-19;
6) Ivermectin leads to far lower case-fatality rates in regions with widespread use

Evidence Base Supporting the Efficacy of Ivermectin in COVID-19 as of January 11, 2021

(RCT's = randomized controlled trials, OCT's = observational controlled trials). Every clinical trial shows a benefit, with RCT's and OCT's reporting the same direction and magnitude; nearly all are statistically significant.

Controlled trials studying the prevention of COVID-19 (8 trials completed)

- 3 RCT's with large statistically significant reductions in transmission rates, a total of 774 patients
- 5 OCT's with large statistically significant reductions in transmission rates, a total of 2,052 patients

Controlled trials in the treatment of both early and hospitalized COVID-19 patients (19 trials completed)

- 5 RCT's with large, significant reductions in time to recovery or hospital length of stay, a total of 774 patients
- 1 RCT with a large, statistically significant reduction in rate of deterioration/hospitalization, total of 363 patients
- 2 RCT's with significant decreases in viral load, days of anosmia, cough, or time to recovery, a total of 85 patients
- 3 RCT's with large, significant reductions in mortality, a total of 695 patients
- 3 OCT's with large, statistically significant reductions in mortality, a total of 1,688 patients

Number of Studies and Patients Among the Existing Clinical Trials of Ivermectin in COVID-19

- 27 controlled trials, including a total of 6,612 patients have been completed using well-matched control groups
- 16 trials, including over 2,500 patients, are prospective, randomized, controlled studies

- 11 of the 27 trials have been published in peer-reviewed journals, 3,900 patients, remainder are in pre-print

Front Line COVID-19 Critical Care Alliance – Recommendation on Ivermectin in COVID-19

Even restricting analysis to just the 16 randomized controlled trials (totaling over 2,500 patients), the majority report a statistically significant reduction in transmission or disease progression or mortality.

Further, a meta-analysis recently performed by an independent research consortium calculated the chances that ivermectin is ineffective in COVID-19 to be 1 in 67 million.

The FLCCC Alliance, based on the totality of the existing evidence, supports an A-I recommendation (NIH rating scheme; strong level, high quality evidence) for the use of ivermectin in both the prophylaxis and treatment of all phases of COVID-19.

Furthermore, we encourage all regulatory agencies to review our manuscript detailing these studies above as well as the multiple population-wide "natural experiments" that occurred in numerous cities and regions after the initiation of ivermectin distribution programs. The widespread use of ivermectin resulted in a significant reduction in cases and mortality rates that approached pre-pandemic levels in these areas. As evidenced by what occurred in these regions, ivermectin is clearly an essential and vital treatment component in achieving control of the pandemic.

In March 2020, the Front Line COVID-19 Critical Care Alliance (FLCCC) was created and led by Professor Paul E. Marik to continuously review the rapidly emerging basic science, translational, and clinical data to develop a treatment protocol for COVID-19. The FLCCC then recently discovered that ivermectin, an anti-parasitic medicine, has highly potent anti-viral and anti-inflammatory properties against COVID-19. They then identified repeated, consistent, large magnitude improvements in clinical outcomes in multiple, large, randomized and observational controlled trials in both prophylaxis and treatment of COVID-19. Further, data showing impacts on population wide health outcomes have resulted from multiple, large "natural experiments" that occurred when various city mayors and regional health ministries within South American countries initiated "ivermectin distribution" campaigns to their citizen populations in the hopes the drug would prove effective.

The tight, reproducible, temporally associated decreases in case counts and case fatality rates in each of those regions compared to nearby regions without such campaigns, suggest that ivermectin may prove to be a global solution to the pandemic. This was further evidenced by the recent incorporation of ivermectin as a prophylaxis and treatment agent for COVID-19 in the national treatment guidelines of Belize, Macedonia, and the state of Uttar Pradesh in Northern India, populated by 210 million people.

To our knowledge, the current review is the earliest to compile sufficient clinical data to demonstrate the strong signal of therapeutic efficacy as it is based on numerous clinical trials in multiple disease phases.

One limitation is that half the controlled trials have been published in peer-reviewed publications, with the remainder taken from manuscripts uploaded to medicine pre-print servers. Although it is now standard practice for trials data from pre-print servers to immediately influence therapeutic practices during the pandemic, given the controversial therapeutics adopted as a result of this practice, the FLCCC argues that it is imperative that our major national and international health care agencies devote the necessary resources to more quickly validate these studies and confirm the major, positive epidemiological impacts that have been recorded when ivermectin is widely distributed among populations with a high incidence of COVID-19 infections.

Pre-Clinical Studies of Ivermectin's activity against SARS-CoV-2

Since 2012, a growing number of cellular studies have demonstrated that ivermectin has anti-viral properties against an increasing number of RNA viruses, including influenza, Zika, HIV, Dengue, and most importantly, SARS-CoV-2 (Mastrangelo et al., 2012; Wagstaff et al., 2012; Tay et al., 2013; Götz et al., 2016; Varghese et al., 2016; Atkinson et al., 2018; Lv et al., 2018; King et al., 2020; Yang et al., 2020).

Insights into the mechanisms of action by which ivermectin both interferes with the entrance and replication of SARS-CoV-2 within human cells are mounting. Caly et al first reported that ivermectin significantly inhibits SARS-CoV-2 replication in a cell culture model, observing the near absence of all viral material 48h after exposure to ivermectin (Caly et al., 2020b).

However, some questioned whether this observation is generalizable clinically given the inability to achieve similar tissue concentrations employed in their experimental model using standard or even massive doses of ivermectin (Bray et al., 2020; Schmith et al., 2020).

It should be noted that the concentrations required for effect in cell culture models bear little resemblance to human physiology given the absence of an active immune system working synergistically with a therapeutic agent such as ivermectin. Further, prolonged durations of exposure to a drug likely would require a fraction of the dosing in short term cell model exposure.

Further, multiple co-existing or alternate mechanisms of action likely explain the clinical effects observed, such as the competitive binding of ivermectin with the host receptor-binding region of

SARS-CoV-2 spike protein, as proposed in six molecular modeling studies (Dayer, 2020; Hussien and Abdelaziz, 2020; Lehrer and Rheinstein, 2020; Maurya, 2020; Nallusamy et al., 2020; Suravajhala et al., 2020).

In four of the studies, ivermectin was identified as having the highest or among the highest of binding affinities to spike protein S1 binding domains of SARS-CoV-2 among hundreds of molecules collectively examined, with ivermectin not being the particular focus of study in four of these studies (Scheim, 2020).

This is the same mechanism by which viral antibodies, in particular, those generated by the Pfizer and Moderna vaccines, contain the SARS-CoV-2 virus.

The high binding activity of ivermectin to the SARS-CoV-2 spike protein could limit binding to either the ACE-2 receptor or sialic acid receptors, respectively either preventing cellular entry of the virus or preventing hemagglutination, a recently proposed pathologic mechanism in COVID-19 (Dasgupta J, 2020; Dayer, 2020; Lehrer and Rheinstein, 2020; Maurya, 2020; Scheim, 2020).

Ivermectin has also been shown to bind to or interfere with multiple essential structural and non-structural proteins required by the virus in order to replicate (Lehrer and Rheinstein, 2020; Sen Gupta et al., 2020).

Finally, ivermectin also binds to the SARS-CoV-2 RNA-dependent RNA polymerase (RdRp), thereby inhibiting viral replication (Swargiary, 2020). Arevalo et al investigated in a murine model infected with a type 2 family RNA coronavirus similar to SARS-CoV-2, (mouse hepatitis virus), the response to 500 mcg/kg of ivermectin vs. placebo (Arevalo et al., 2020).

The study included 40 infected mice, with 20 treated with ivermectin, 20 with phosphate buffered saline, and then 16 uninfected control mice that were also given phosphate buffered saline.

At day 5, all the mice were euthanized to obtain tissues for examination and viral load assessment.

The 20 non-ivermectin treated infected mice all showed severe hepatocellular necrosis surrounded by a severe lymphoplasmacytic inflammatory infiltration associated with a high hepatic viral load (52,158 AU), while in the ivermectin treated mice a much lower viral load was measured (23,192 AU; $p<0.05$), with only few livers in the ivermectin treated mice showing histopathological damage such that the differences between the livers from the uninfected control mice were not statistically significant.

Dias De Melo and colleagues recently posted the results of a study they did with golden hamsters that were intranasally inoculated with SARS-CoV-2 virus, and at the time of the infection, the animals also received a single subcutaneous injection of ivermectin at a dose of 0.4mg/kg on day 1 (de Melo et al., 2020).

Control animals received only the physiologic solution. They found the following among the ivermectin treated hamsters; a dramatic reduction in anosmia (33.3% vs 83.3%, $p=.03$) which was also sex-dependent in that the male hamsters exhibited a reduction in clinical score while the treated female hamsters failed to show any sign of anosmia.

They also found significant reductions in cytokine concentrations in the nasal turbinate's and lungs of the treated animals despite the lack of apparent differences in viral titers.

Despite these mounting insights into the existing and potential mechanisms of action of ivermectin both as a prophylactic and treatment agent, it must be emphasized that significant research gaps remain and that many further in vitro and animal studies should be undertaken to better define not only these mechanisms but also to further support ivermectin's role as a prophylactic agent, especially in terms of the optimal dose and frequency required.

Pre-Clinical studies of ivermectin's anti-inflammatory properties

Given that little viral replication occurs in the later phases of COVID-19, nor can virus be cultured, and only in a minority of autopsies can viral cytopathic changes be found (Perera et al., 2020; Polak et al., 2020;Young et al., 2020), the most likely pathophysiologic mechanism is that identified by Li et al. where they showed that the non-viable RNA fragments of SARS-CoV-2 leads to a high mortality and morbidity in COVID-19 via the provocation of an overwhelming and injurious inflammatory response (Li et al., 2013).

Based on these insights and the clinical benefits of ivermectin in late phase disease to be reviewed below, it appears that the increasingly well described in vitro properties of ivermectin as an inhibitor of inflammation are far more clinically potent than previously recognized.

The growing list of studies demonstrating the anti-inflammatory properties of ivermectin include its ability to; inhibit cytokine production after lipopolysaccharide exposure, downregulate transcription of NF-kB, and limit the production of both nitric oxide and prostaglandin E2 (Zhang et al., 2008;Ci et al., 2009;Zhang et al., 2009).

Exposure prophylaxis studies of ivermectin's ability to prevent transmission of COVID-19

Data is also now available showing large and statistically significant decreases in the transmission of COVID-19 among human subjects based on data from three randomized controlled trials (RCT) and five observational controlled trials (OCT) with four of the eight (two of them RCT's) published in peer-reviewed journals (Behera et al., 2020; Bernigaud et al., 2020; Carvallo et al., 2020b; Chala, 2020; Elgazzar et al., 2020; Hellwig and Maia, 2020; Shouman, 2020).

Elgazzar and colleagues at Benha University in Egypt randomized 200 health care and households contacts of COVID-19 patients where the intervention group consisted of 100 patients given a high dose of 0.4mg/kg on day 1 and a second dose on day 7 in addition to wearing personal protective equipment (PPE), while the control group of 100 contacts wore PPE only (Elgazzar et al., 2020).

They reported a large and statistically significant reduction in contacts testing positive by RTPCR when treated with ivermectin vs. controls, 2% vs 10%, $p<.05$. Shouman conducted an RCT at Zagazig University in Egypt, including 340 (228 treated, 112 control) family members of patients positive for SARS-CoV-2 via PCR (Shouman, 2020). Ivermectin, (approximately 0.25mg/kg) was administered twice, on the day of the positive test and 72 hours later.

After a two-week follow up, a large and statistically significant decrease in COVID-19 symptoms among household members treated with ivermectin was found, 7.4% vs. 58.4%, $p<.001$.

Recently Alam et al from Bangladesh performed a prospective observational study of 118 patients that were evenly split into those that volunteered for either the treatment or control arms, described as a persuasive approach. Although this method, along with the study being unblinded likely led to confounders, the differences between the two groups were so large (6.7% vs. 73.3%, p<.001) and similar to the other prophylaxis trial results that confounders alone are unlikely to explain such a result (Alam et al., 2020).

Carvallo et al also performed a prospective observational trial where they gave healthy volunteers ivermectin and carrageenan daily for 28 days and matched them to similarly healthy controls who did not take the medicines (Carvallo et al., 2020b).

Of the 229 study subjects, 131 were treated with 0.2mg of ivermectin drops taken by mouth five times per day. After 28 days, none of those receiving ivermectin prophylaxis group had tested positive for SARS-COV-2 versus 11.2% of patients in the control arm (p<.001).

In a much larger follow-up observational controlled trial by the same group that included 1,195 health care workers, they found that over a 3-month period, there were no infections recorded among the 788 workers that took weekly ivermectin prophylaxis while 58% of the 407 controls had become ill with COVID-19.

This study demonstrates that protection against transmission can be achieved among high-risk health care workers by taking 12mg once weekly (Carvallo et al., 2020b). The Carvallo IVERCAR protocol was also separately tested in a prospective RCT by the Health Ministry of Tucuman, Argentina where they found that among 234 health care workers, the intervention group that took 12 mg once weekly, only 3.4% contracted COVID-19 vs. 21.4% of controls, p<.0001(Chala, 2020).

The need for weekly dosing in the Carvallo study over a 4-month period may not have been necessary given that, in a recent RCT from Dhaka, Bangladesh, the intervention group (n=58) took 12mg only once monthly for a similar 4-month period and also reported a large and statistically significant decrease in infections compared to controls, 6.9% vs. 73.3%, $p<.05$ (Alam et al., 2020).

Then, in a large retrospective observational case-control study from India, Behera et al. reported that among 186 case-control pairs (n=372) of health care workers, they identified 169 participants that had taken some form of prophylaxis, with 115 that had taken ivermectin prophylaxis (Behera et al., 2020).

After matched pair analysis, they reported that in the workers who had taken two dose ivermectin prophylaxis, the odds ratio for contracting COVID-19 was markedly decreased (0.27, 95% CI, 0.15–0.51). Notably, one dose prophylaxis was not found to be protective in this study. Based on both their study finding and the Egyptian prophylaxis study, the All-India Institute of Medical Sciences instituted a prophylaxis protocol for their health care workers where they now take two 0.3mg/kg doses of ivermectin 72 hours apart and repeat the dose monthly.

Data which further illuminates the protective role of ivermectin against COVID-19 comes from a study of nursing home residents in France which reported that in a facility that suffered a scabies outbreak where all 69 residents and 52 staff were treated with ivermectin (Behera et al., 2020), they found that during the time period surrounding this event, 7/69 residents fell ill with COVID-19 (10.1%).

In this group with an average age of 90 years, only one resident required oxygen support and no resident died. In a matched control group of residents from surrounding facilities, they found 22.6% of residents fell ill and 4.9% died. Likely the most definitive evidence supporting the efficacy of ivermectin as a prophylaxis agent was published recently in the International Journal of Anti-

Microbial agents where a group of researchers analyzed data using the prophylactic chemotherapy databank administered by the WHO along with case counts obtained by Worldometers, a public data aggregation site used by among others, the Johns Hopkins University (Hellwig and Maia, 2020).

When they compared the data from countries with active ivermectin mass drug administration programs for the prevention of parasite infections, they discovered that the COVID-19 case counts were significantly lower in the countries with recently active programs, to a high degree of statistical significance, $p<.001$.

Further data supporting a role for ivermectin in decreasing transmission rates can be found from South American countries where, in retrospect, large "natural experiments" appear to have occurred.

For instance, beginning as early as May, various regional health ministries and governmental authorities within Peru, Brazil, and Paraguay initiated "ivermectin distribution" campaigns to their citizen populations (Chamie, 2020).

In one such example from Brazil, the cities of Itajai, Macapa, and Natal distributed massive amounts of ivermectin doses to their city's population, where, in the case of Natal, 1 million doses were distributed. The distribution campaign of Itajai began in mid-July, and in Natal they began on June 30th , and in Macapa, the capital city of Amapa and others nearby incorporated ivermectin into their treatment protocols in late May after they were particularly hard hit in April.

Clinical studies on the efficacy of Ivermectin in treating mildly ill outpatients

Currently, seven trials which include a total of over 3,000 patients with mild outpatient illness have been completed, a set comprised of 7 RCT's and four case series (Babalola et al.; Cadegiani et al., 2020; Carvallo et al., 2020a; Chaccour et al., 2020; Chowdhury et al., 2020; Espitia-Hernandez et al., 2020; Gorial et al., 2020; Hashim et al., 2020; Khan et al., 2020; Mahmud, 2020; Podder et al., 2020; Ravikirti et al., 2021).

The largest, a double blinded RCT by Mahmud et al. was conducted in Dhaka, Bangladesh and targeted 400 patients with 363 patients completing the study (Mahmud, 2020).

In this study, as in many other of the clinical studies to be reviewed, either a tetracycline (doxycycline) or macrolide antibiotic (azithromycin) was included as part of the treatment. The importance of including antibiotics such as doxycycline or azithromycin is unclear, however, both tetracycline and macrolide Antibiotics have recognized anti-inflammatory, immunomodulatory, and even antiviral effects.

Although the posted data from this study does not specify the amount of mildly ill outpatients vs. hospitalized patients treated, important clinical outcomes were profoundly impacted, with increased rates of early improvement (60.7% vs. 44.4% p<.03) and decreased rates of clinical deterioration (8.7% vs 17.8%, p<.02). Given that mildly ill outpatients mainly comprised the study cohort, only two deaths were observed (both in the control group). Ravikirti performed a double-blind RCT of 115 patients, ang although the primary outcome of PCR positivity on Day 6 was no different, the secondary outcome of mortality was 0%vs. 6.9%, p=.019 (Ravikirti et al., 2021). Babalola in Nigeria also performed a double blind-RCT of 62 patients, and, in contrast to Ravikirti, they found a significant difference in viral clearance between both the low and high dose treatment groups and controls in a dose dependent fashion, p=.006 (Babalola et al.).

Another RCT by Hashim et al. in Baghdad, Iraq included 140 patients equally divided; the control group received standard care, the treated group included a combination of both outpatient and hospitalized patients (Hashim et al., 2020). In the 96 patients with mild-to-moderate outpatient illness, they treated 48 patients with a combination of ivermectin/doxycycline and standard of care and compared outcomes to the 48 patients treated with standard of care alone.

The standard of care in this trial included many elements of the MATH+ protocol, such as dexamethasone 6mg/day or methylprednisolone 40mg twice per day if needed, Vitamin C 1000mg twice/day, Zinc 75–125mg/day, Vitamin D3 5000 IU/day, azithromycin 250mg/day for 5 days, and acetaminophen 500mg as needed.

Although no patients in either group progressed or died, the time to recovery was significantly shorter in the ivermectin treated group (6.3 days vs 13.7 days, p<.0001).

Chaccour et al conducted a small, double-blinded RCT in Spain where they randomized 24 patients to ivermectin vs placebo and although they found no difference in PCR positivity at day 7, they did find statistically significant decreases in viral loads, patient days of anosmia (76 vs 158, p<.05), and patient days with cough (68 vs 98, p<.05) (Chaccour et al., 2020).

Another RCT of ivermectin treatment in 116 outpatients was performed by Chowdhury et al. in Bangladesh where they compared a group of 60 patients treated with the combination of ivermectin/ doxycycline to a group of 60 patients treated with hydroxychloroquine/doxycycline with a primary outcome of time to negative PCR (Chowdhury et al., 2020). Although they found no difference in this outcome, in the treatment group, the time to symptomatic recovery approached statistical significance (5.9 days vs. 7.0 days, p=.07). In another smaller RCT of 62 patients by Podder et al., they also found a shorter time to symptomatic recovery that approached statistical significance (10.1 days vs 11.5 days, p>.05, 95% CI, 0.86–3.67) (Podder et al., 2020).

A medical group in the Dominican Republic reported a case series of 2,688 consecutive symptomatic outpatients seeking treatment in the emergency room, the majority of whom were diagnosed using a clinical algorithm. The patients were treated with high dose ivermectin of 0.4mg/kg for one dose along with five days of azithromycin. Only 16 of the 2,688 patients (0.59%) required subsequent hospitalization with one death recorded (Morgenstern et al., 2020).

In another case series of 100 patients in Bangladesh, all treated with a combination of 0.2mg/kg ivermectin and doxycycline, they found that no patient required hospitalization nor died, and all patients' symptoms improved within 72 hours (Robin et al., 2020).

A case series from Argentina reported on a combination protocol which used ivermectin, aspirin, dexamethasone and enoxaparin. In the 135 mild illness patients, all survived (Carvallo et al., 2020a). Similarly, a case series from Mexico of 28 consecutively treated patients with ivermectin, all were reported to have recovered with an average time to full recovery of only 3.6 days (Espitia Hernandez et al., 2020).

Clinical studies of the efficacy of ivermectin in hospitalized patients

Studies of ivermectin amongst more severely ill hospitalized patients include 6 RCT's, 5 OCTs, and a database analysis study (Ahmed et al., 2020; Budhiraja et al., 2020; Camprubi et al., 2020; Chachar et al., 2020; Elgazzar et al., 2020; Gorial et al., 2020; Hashim et al., 2020; Khan et al., 2020; Niaee et al., 2020; Portmann-Baracco et al., 2020; Rajter et al., 2020; Soto-Becerra et al., 2020; Spoorthi V, 2020).

The largest RCT in hospitalized patients was performed concurrent with the prophylaxis study reviewed above by Elgazzar et al (Elgazzar et al., 2020). 400 patients were randomized amongst 4 treatment groups of 100 patients each. Groups 1 and 2 included mild/moderate illness patients only, with Group 1 treated with one dose 0.4mg/kg ivermectin plus standard of care (SOC) and Group 2 received hydroxychloroquine (HCQ) 400mg twice on day 1 then 200mg twice daily for 5 days plus standard of care.

There was a statistically significant lower rate of progression in the ivermectin treated group (1% vs. 22%, p<.001) with no deaths and 4 deaths respectively. Groups 3 and 4 all included only severely ill patients, with group 3 again treated with single dose of 0.4mg/kg plus SOC while Group 4 received HCQ plus SOC. In this severely ill subgroup, the differences in outcomes were even larger, with lower rates of progression 4% vs. 30%, and mortality 2% vs 20% (p<.001).

The one largely outpatient RCT done by Hashim reviewed above also included 22 hospitalized patients in each group. In the ivermectin/doxycycline treated group, there were 11 severely ill patients and 11 critically ill patients while in the standard care group, only severely ill patients (n=22) were included due to their ethical concerns of including critically ill patients in the control group (45).

This decision led to a marked imbalance in the severity of illness between these hospitalized patient groups. However, despite the mismatched severity of illness between groups and the small number of patients included, beneficial differences in outcomes were seen, but not all reached statistical significance. For instance, there was a large reduction in the rate of progression of illness (9% vs. 31.8%, p=0.15) and, most importantly, there was a large difference in mortality amongst the severely ill groups which reached a borderline statistical significance, (0% vs 27.3%, p=.052). Another important finding was the surprisingly low mortality rate of 18% found among the subset of critically ill patients, all of whom were treated with ivermectin.

A recent RCT from Iran found a dramatic reduction in mortality with ivermectin use (Niaee et al., 2020). Among multiple ivermectin treatment arms (different ivermectin dosing strategies were used in the intervention arms), the average mortality was reported as 3.3% while the average mortality within the standard care and placebo arms was 18.8%, with an OR of 0.18 (95% CI 0.06-0.55, p<.05).

Spoorthi and Sasanak performed a prospective RCT of 100 hospitalized patients whereby they treated 50 with ivermectin and doxycycline while the 50 controls were given a placebo consisting of Vitamin B6 (Spoorthi V, 2020). Although no deaths were reported in either group, the ivermectin treatment group had a shorter hospital LOS 3.7 days vs 4.7 days, p=.03, and a shorter time to complete resolution of symptoms, 6.7 days vs 7.9 days, p=.01.

The largest OCT (n=280) in hospitalized patients was done by Rajter et al. at Broward Health Hospitals in Florida and was recently published in the major medical journal Chest (43). They performed a retrospective OCT with a propensity matched design on 280 consecutive treated patients and compared those treated with ivermectin to those without. 173 patients were treated with ivermectin (160 received a single dose, 13 received a 2nd dose at day 7) while 107 were not (Rajter et al., 2020).

In both unmatched and propensity matched cohort comparisons, similar, large, and statistically significant lower mortality was found amongst ivermectin treated patients (15.0% vs. 25.2%, p=.03).

Further, in the subgroup of patients with severe pulmonary involvement, mortality was profoundly reduced when treated with ivermectin (38.8% vs. 80.7%, p=.001).

Another large OCT in Bangladesh compared 115 pts treated with ivermectin to a standard care cohort consisting of 133 patients (Khan et al., 2020). Despite a significantly higher proportion of patients in the ivermectin group being male (i.e., with well-described, lower survival rates in COVID), the groups were otherwise well matched, yet the mortality decrease was statistically significant (0.9% vs. 6.8%, p<.05).

The largest OCT is a study from Brazil which included almost 1,500 patients (Portmann Baracco et al., 2020). Although the primary data was not provided, they reported that in 704 hospitalized patients treated with a single dose of 0.15mg/kg ivermectin compared to 704 controls, overall mortality was reduced (1.4% vs. 8.5%, HR 0.2, 95% CI 0.12-0.37, p<.0001). Similarly, in the patients on mechanical ventilation, mortality was also reduced (1.3% vs. 7.3%).

A small study from Baghdad, Iraq compared 16 ivermectin treated patients to 71 controls (Gorial et al., 2020). This study also reported a significant reduction in length of hospital stay (7.6 days vs. 13.2 days, p<.001) in the ivermectin group.

In a study reporting on the first 1000 patients treated in a hospital in India, they found that in the 34 patients treated with ivermectin alone, all recovered and were discharged, while in the over 900 patients treated with other agents, there was an overall mortality of 11.1% (Budhiraja et al., 2020).

One retrospective analysis of a database of hospitalized patients compared responses in patients receiving ivermectin, azithromycin, hydroxychloroquine or combinations of these medicines.

In this study, no benefit for ivermectin was found, however the treatment groups in this analysis all included a number of patients who died on day 2, while in the control groups no early deaths occurred, thus the comparison appears limited (Soto-Becerra et al., 2020).

Meta-analyses of the above controlled treatment trials were performed by the study authors focused on the two important clinical outcomes: time to clinical recovery and mortality. The consistent and reproducible signals leading to large overall statistically significant benefits from within both study designs is remarkable, especially given that in several of the studies treatment was initiated late in the disease course.

Ivermectin in post-COVID-19 syndrome

Increasing reports of persistent, vexing, and even disabling symptoms after recovery from acute COVID-19 have been reported and which many have termed the condition as "long Covid" and patients as "long haulers", estimated to occur in approximately 10% of cases (Callard and Perego, 2020; Rubin, 2020; Siegelman, 2020).

Generally considered as a post-viral syndrome consisting of a chronic and sometimes disabling constellation of symptoms which include, in order, fatigue, shortness of breath, joint pains and chest pain. Many patients describe their most disabling symptom as impaired memory and concentration, often with extreme fatigue, described as "brain fog", and are highly suggestive of the condition myalgic encephalomyelitis/chronic fatigue syndrome, a condition well reported to begin after viral infections, in particular with Epstein-Barr virus.

Although no specific treatments have been identified for long COVID, a recent manuscript by Aguirre-Chang et al from the National University of San Marcos in Peru reported on the experience with ivermectin in such patients (Aguirre-Chang, 2020).

They treated 33 patients who were between 4 and 12 weeks from the onset of symptoms with escalating doses of ivermectin; 0.2mg/kg for 2 days if mild, 0.4mg/kg for 2 days if moderate, with doses extended if symptoms persisted. They found that in 87.9% of the patients, resolution of all symptoms was observed after two doses with an additional 7% reporting complete resolution after additional doses. Their experience suggests the need for controlled studies to better test efficacy in this vexing syndrome.

Safety of Ivermectin

Numerous studies report low rates of adverse events, with the majority mild, transient, and largely attributed to the body's inflammatory response to the death of the parasites and include itching, rash, swollen lymph nodes, joint paints, fever and headache (Kircik et al., 2016).

In a study which combined results from trials including over 50,000 patients, serious events occurred in less than 1% and largely associated with administration in Loa loa (Gardon et al., 1997).

Further, according to the pharmaceutical reference standard Lexicomp, the only medications contraindicated for use with ivermectin are the concurrent administration of anti-tuberculosis and cholera vaccines while the anticoagulant warfarin would require dose monitoring.

Another special caution is that immunosuppressed or organ transplant patients who are on calcineurin inhibitors such as tacrolimus or cyclosporine or the immunosuppressant sirolimus should have close monitoring of drug levels when on ivermectin given that interactions exist which can affect these levels. A longer list of drug interactions can be found on the **drugs.com** database, with nearly all interactions leading to a possibility of either increased or decreased blood levels of ivermectin. Given studies showing tolerance and lack of adverse effects in human subjects given escalating high doses of ivermectin, toxicity is unlikely although a reduced efficacy due to decreased levels may be a concern (Guzzo et al., 2002).

Concerns of safety in the setting of liver disease are unfounded given that, to our knowledge, only two cases of liver injury have ever been reported in association with ivermectin, with both cases rapidly resolved without need for treatment. (Sparsa et al., 2006;

Veit et al., 2006). Further, no dose adjustments are required in patients with liver disease. Some have described ivermectin as potentially neurotoxic, yet one study performed a search of a global pharmaceutical database and found only 28 cases of serious neurological adverse events such as ataxia, altered consciousness, seizure, or tremor (Chandler, 2018).

Potential explanations included the effects of concomitantly administered drugs which increase absorption past the blood brain barrier or polymorphisms in the mdr-1 gene. However, the total number of reported cases suggests that such events are rare. Finally, ivermectin has been used safely in pregnant women, children, and infants.

Currently, as of December 14, 2020, the accumulating evidence demonstrating the safety and efficacy of ivermectin in COVID-19 strongly supports its immediate use on a risk/benefit calculation in the context of a pandemic. Large-scale epidemiologic analyses validate the findings of in vitro, animal, prophylaxis, and clinical studies. Regions of the world with widespread ivermectin use have demonstrated a sizable reduction in case counts, hospitalizations, and fatality rates.

This approach should be urgently considered in the presence of an escalating COVID-19 pandemic and as a bridge to vaccination. A recent systematic review of eight RCTs by Australian researchers, published as a preprint, similarly concluded that ivermectin treatment led to a reduction in mortality, time to clinical recovery, the incidence of disease progression, and duration of hospital admission in patients across all stages of clinical severity (Kalfas et al., 2020). Our current review includes a total of 6,612 patients from 27 controlled studies [16 of them were RCTs, 5 double blinded, one single blinded, (n= 2,503)]; 11 published in peer-reviewed journals including 3,900 patients.

Pre-print publications have exploded during the COVID-19 pandemic.

Except for hydroxychloroquine and convalescent plasma that were widely adopted before availability of any clinical data to support, almost all subsequent therapeutics were adopted after pre-print publication and prior to peer review. Examples include remdesivir, corticosteroids, and monoclonal antibodies.

An even more aggressive example of rapid adoption was the initiation of inoculation programs using novel mRNA vaccines prior to review of either pre-print or peer-reviewed trials data by physicians ordering the inoculations for patients.

In all such situations, both academia and governmental health care agencies relaxed their standard to rise to the needs dictated by the pandemic.

In the context of ivermectin's long standing safety record, low cost, and wide availability along with the consistent, reproducible, large magnitude findings on transmission rates, need for hospitalization, mortality, and population-wide control of COVID-19 case and fatality rates in areas with widespread ivermectin distribution, insisting on the remaining studies to pass peer review prior to widespread adoption appears to be imprudent and to deviate from the now established standard approach towards adoption of new therapeutics during the pandemic. In fact, insisting on such a barrier to adoption would actually violate this new standard given that 12 of the 24 controlled trials have already been published in peer reviewed journals.

In regard to concerns over the validity of observational trial findings, it must be recognized that in the case of ivermectin; 1) half of the trials employed a randomized, controlled trial design (12 of the 24 reviewed above), and 2) that observational and randomized trial designs reach equivalent conclusions on average in nearly all diseases studied, as reported in a large Cochrane review of the topic from 2014 (Anglemyer et al., 2014). In particular, OCTs that employ propensity-matching techniques (as in the Rajter study from Florida), find near identical conclusions to later-conducted RCTs in many different disease states, including coronary syndromes, critical illness, and surgery (Dahabreh et al., 2012; Lonjon et al., 2014; Kitsios et al., 2015). Similarly, as evidenced in the prophylaxis and treatment trial meta-analyses as well as the summary trials table, the entirety of the benefits found in both OCT and RCT trial designs align in both direction and magnitude of benefit.

Such a consistency of benefit amongst numerous trials of varying designs from multiple different countries and centers around the world is both unique in the history of evidence-based medicine and provides strong, additional support to the conclusions reached in this review.

All must consider Declaration 37 of the World Medical Association's "Helsinki Declaration on the Ethical Principles for Medical Research Involving Human Subjects," first established in 1964, which states:

In the treatment of an individual patient, where proven interventions do not exist or other known interventions have been ineffective, the physician, after seeking expert advice, with informed consent from the patient or a legally authorized representative, may use an unproven intervention if in the physician's judgement it offers hope of saving life, re-establishing health or alleviating suffering. This intervention should subsequently be made the object of research, designed to evaluate its safety and efficacy. In all cases, new information must be recorded and, where appropriate, made publicly available.

The continued challenges faced by health care providers in deciding on appropriate therapeutic interventions in patients with COVID-19 would be greatly eased if more updated and definitive evidence-based guidance came from the leading governmental health care agencies. Currently, in the United States, the treatment guidelines for COVID-19 are issued by the National Institutes of Health (NIH).

Unfortunately, the NIH's recommendation on the use of ivermectin in COVID-19 patients was last updated on August 27, 2020. At that time, ivermectin received a recommendation of A-III against use outside of a clinical trial. An A-III recommendation, per the NIH recommendation scheme, means that it was a strong opinion (A), and based on expert opinion only (III) given that presumably little clinical evidence existed at the time to otherwise inform that recommendation.

Based on the totality of the clinical and epidemiologic evidence presented in this review, and in the context of a worsening pandemic in parts of the globe where ivermectin is not widely used, the authors believe the recommendation must be immediately updated to support and guide the nation's health care providers. One aspect that the NIH expert panel may debate is on the grade of recommendation that should be assigned to ivermectin. Based on the NIH rating scheme, the strongest recommendation possible would be an A-I in support of ivermectin which requires "one or more randomized trials with clinical outcomes and/or laboratory endpoints." Given that data from 16 randomized controlled trials (RCT's) demonstrate consistent and large improvements in "clinical outcomes" such as transmission rates, hospitalization rates, and death rates, it appears that the criteria for an A-I level recommendation has been exceeded.

However, although troubling to consider, if experts somehow conclude that the entirety of the available RCT data should be invalidated and dismissed given that either; they were conducted outside of US shores and not by US pharmaceutical companies or academic research centers, that some studies were small or of "low quality", or that such data from foreign countries are not generalizable to American patients, an A-II level recommendation would then have to be considered. In the context of worsening pandemic conditions, when considering a safe, low-cost, widely available early treatment option, even an A-II would result in immediate, widespread adoption by providers in the treatment of COVID-19.

The criteria for an A-II requires supportive findings from "one of more well-designed non-randomized, or observational cohort studies". Fortunately, there are many such studies on ivermectin in COVID-19, with one of the largest and best designed being Dr. Rajter's study from Florida, published in the major peer-reviewed medical journal Chest, where they used propensity matching, a technique accorded by many to be as valid a design as RCT's. Thus, at a minimum, an A-II recommendation is met, which again would and should lead to immediate and widespread adoption in early outpatient treatment, an area that has been little investigated and is devoid of any highly effective therapies at the time of this writing.

Further, it is clear that these data presented far exceed any other NIH strength or quality level such as moderate strength (B), weak strength (C) or grade III quality. To merit the issuance of these lower grades of recommendation would require both a dismissal of the near entirety of the evidence presented in this review in addition to a risk benefit calculation resulting in the belief that the risks of widespread ivermectin use would far exceed any possible benefits in the context of rising case counts, deaths, lockdowns, unemployment, evictions, and bankruptcies.

It is the authors opinion, that based on the totality of these data, the use of ivermectin as a prophylactic and early treatment option should receive an A-I level recommendation by the NIH in support of use by the nation's health care providers.

When, or if, such a recommendation is issued, the Front Line COVID-19 Critical Care Alliance has developed a prophylaxis and early treatment protocol for COVID-19 (I-MASK+), centered around ivermectin combined with masking, social distancing, hand hygiene, Vitamin D, Vitamin C, quercetin, melatonin, and zinc, with all components known for either their anti-viral, anti-inflammatory, or preventive actions. The I-MASK+ protocol suggests treatment approaches for prophylaxis of high-risk patients, post-exposure prophylaxis of household members with COVID-19, and an early treatment approach for patients ill with COVID-19.

In summary, based on the existing and cumulative body of evidence, we recommend the use of ivermectin in both prophylaxis and treatment for COVID-19. In the presence of a global COVID-19 surge, the widespread use of this safe, inexpensive, and effective intervention would lead to a drastic reduction in transmission rates and the morbidity and mortality in mild, moderate, and even severe disease phases. The authors are encouraged and hopeful at the prospect of the many favorable public health and societal impacts that would result once adopted for use.